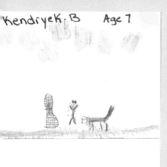
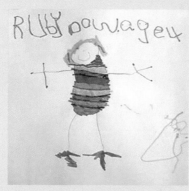
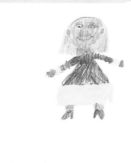

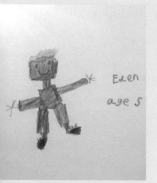
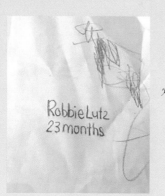
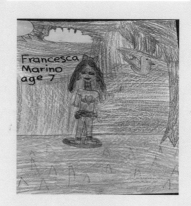
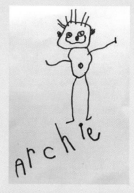
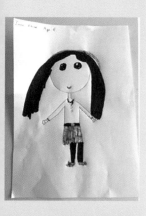
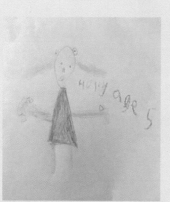
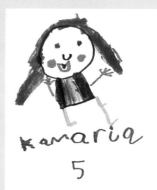
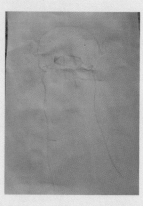
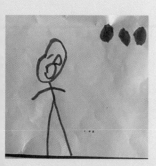
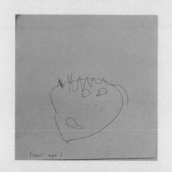

We have allergies too

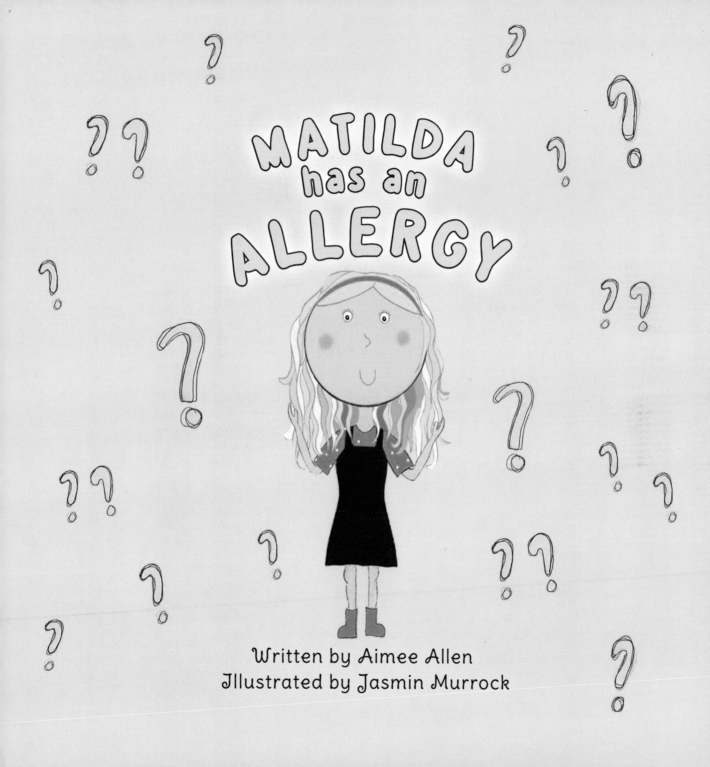

MATILDA has an ALLERGY

Written by Aimee Allen
Illustrated by Jasmin Murrock

ISBN: 978-1-78324-157-6

Published by Wordzworth
www.wordzworth.com

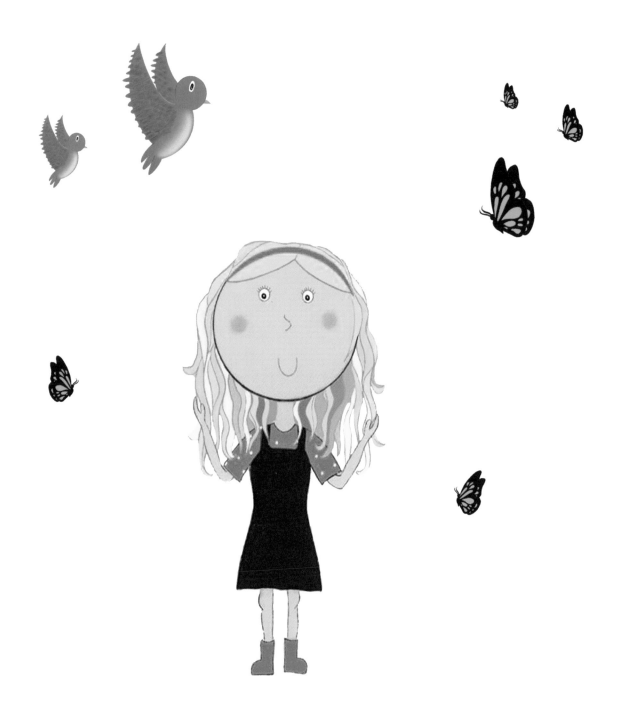

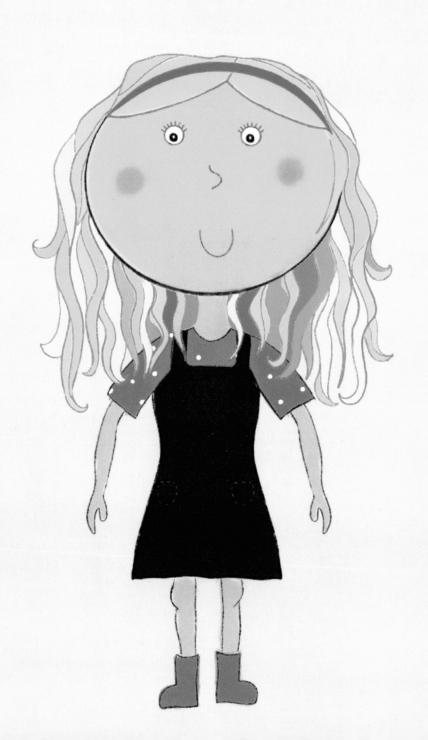

This is Matilda. She is 5 years old and has sunshine coloured hair. Matilda loves being Matilda

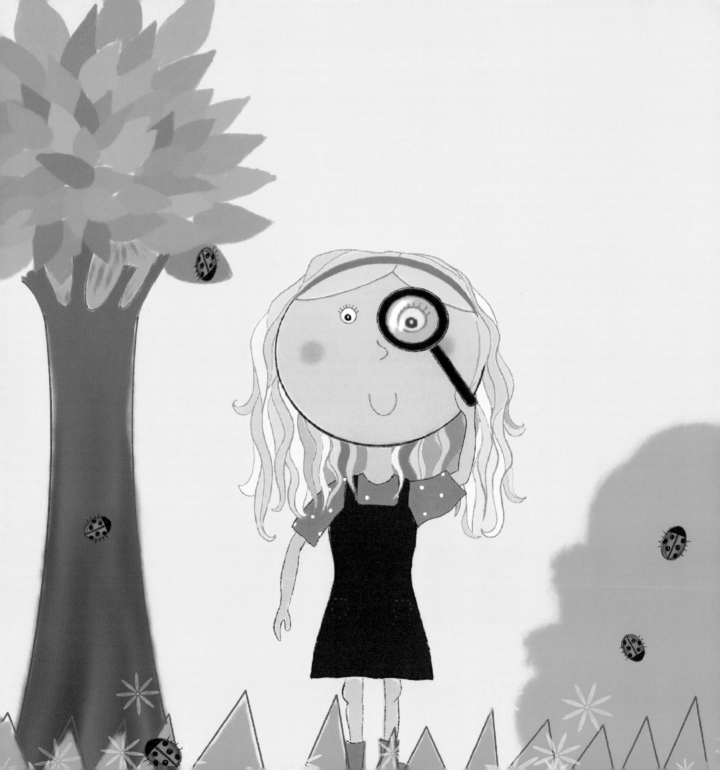

There are many things that Matilda likes to do. She loves to look for creepy crawly creatures in her garden

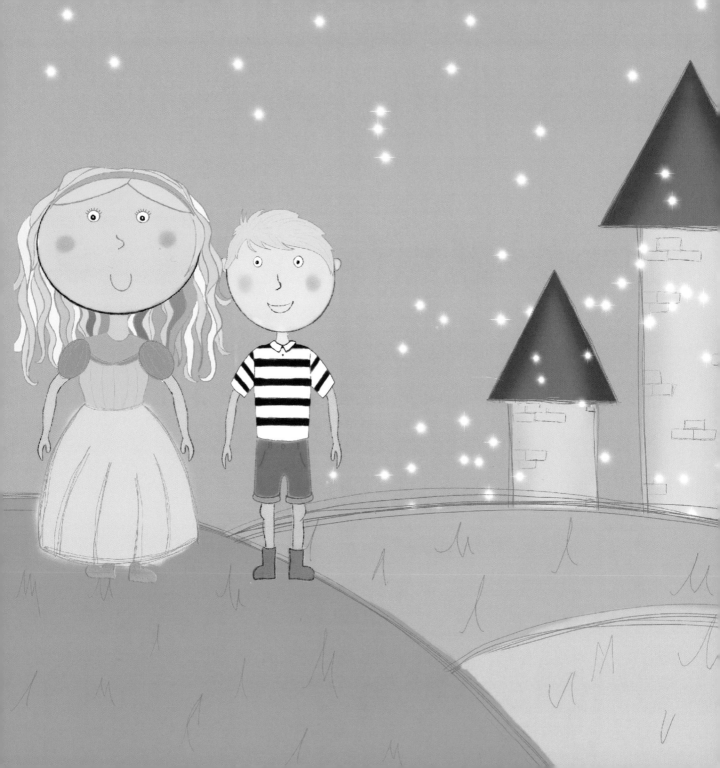

With her brother George, she loves to escape to faraway lands with majestic castles and twinkly stars

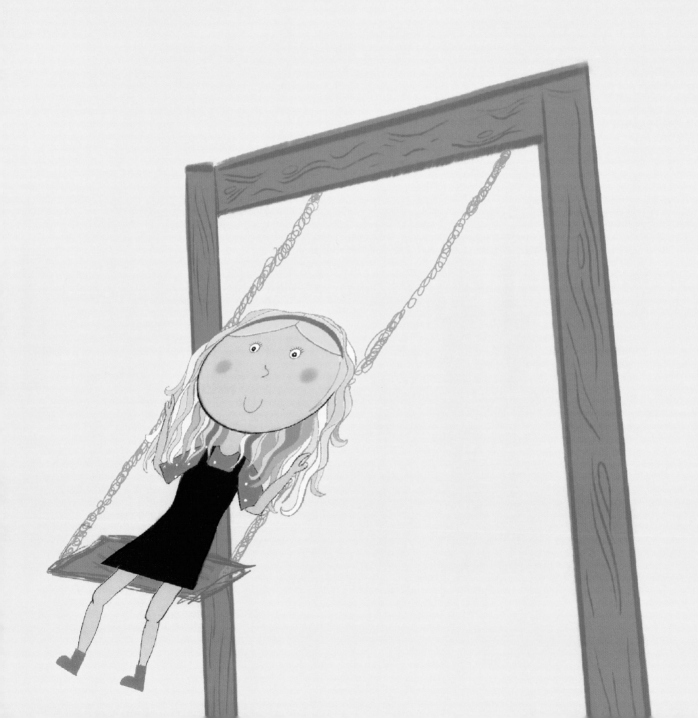

Matilda loves to swing as high as the sky

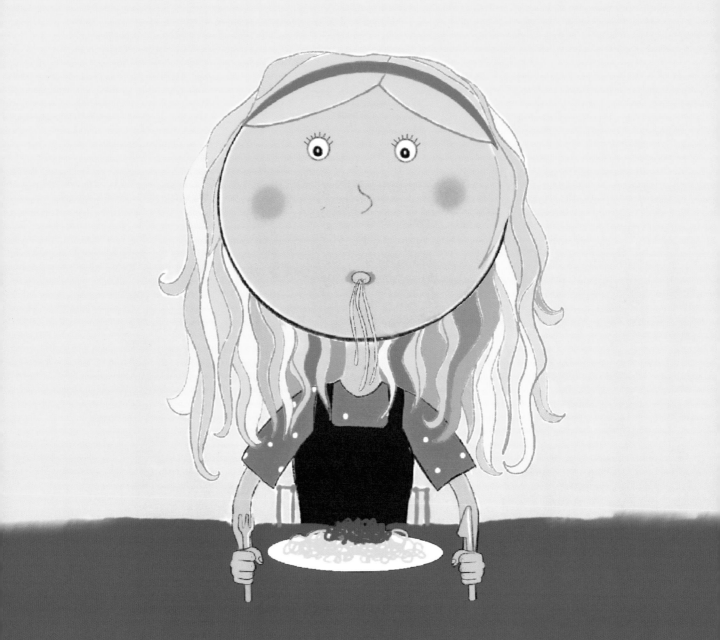

And her most favourite food ever is spaghetti bolognese

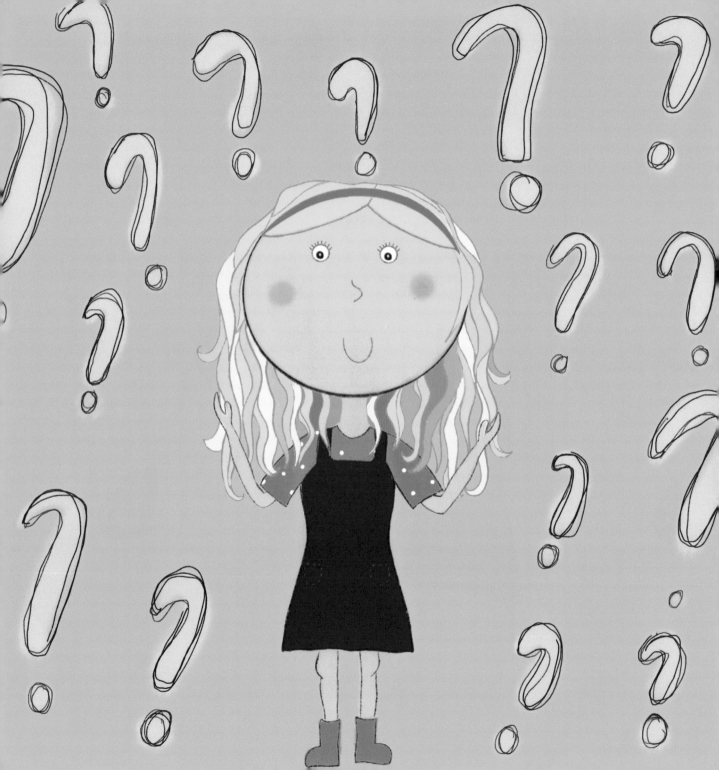

There's also something extra special about Matilda...

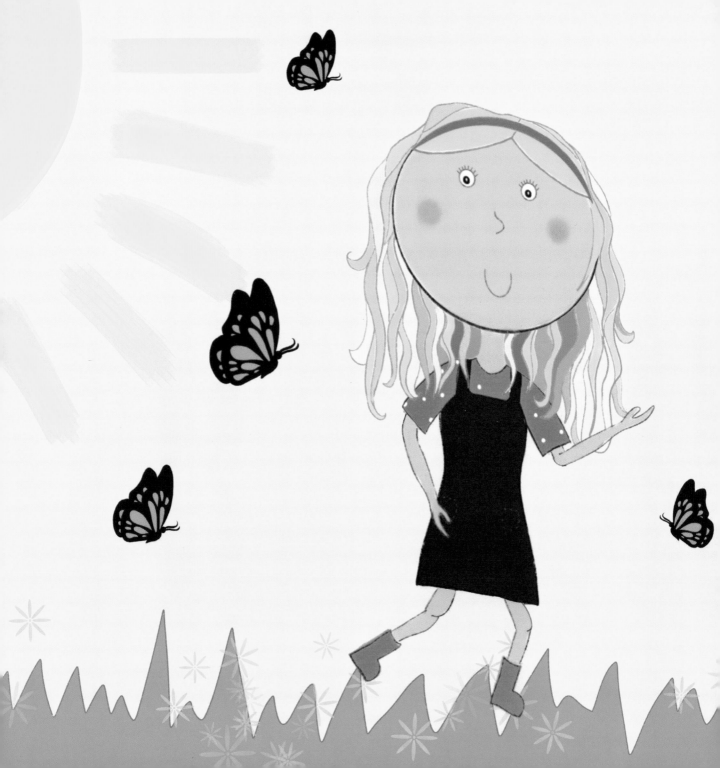

Matilda has an allergy.

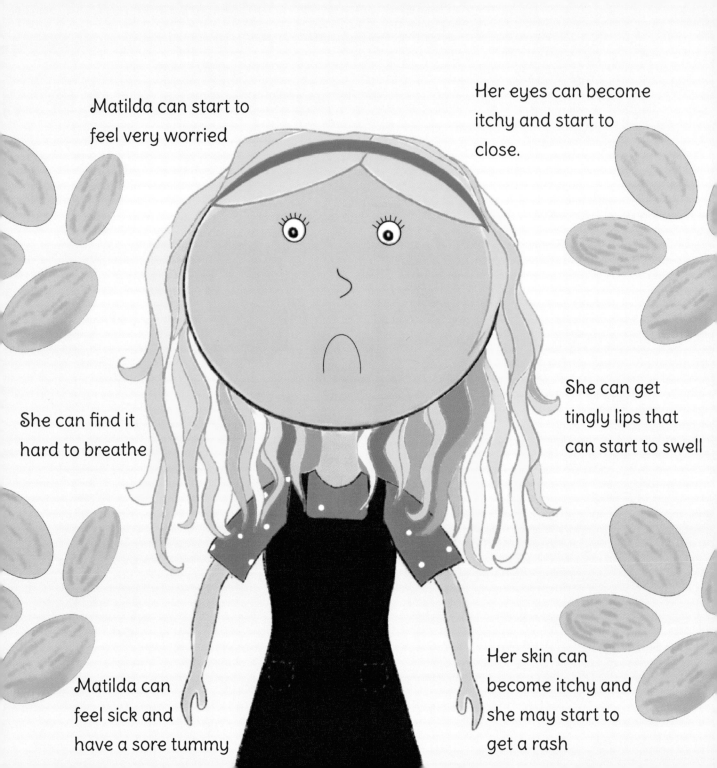

Matilda is allergic to nuts. This means Matilda's body does not like nuts. If she eats a nut she can become very poorly.

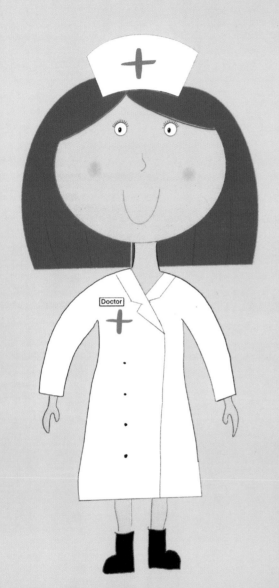

Doctor

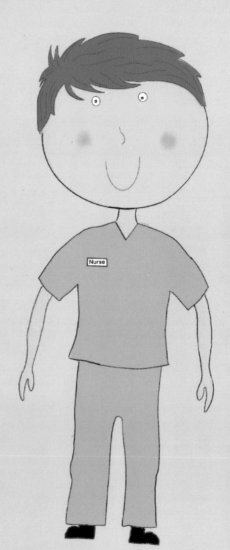

Nurse

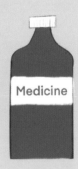

Medicine

Auto-injector

The doctors and nurses have given Matilda
some medicine and a special type of pen
with a needle in. This pen can be used
to give Matilda an injection if she ever
accidentally eats a nut.

There are many things people can be allergic to including

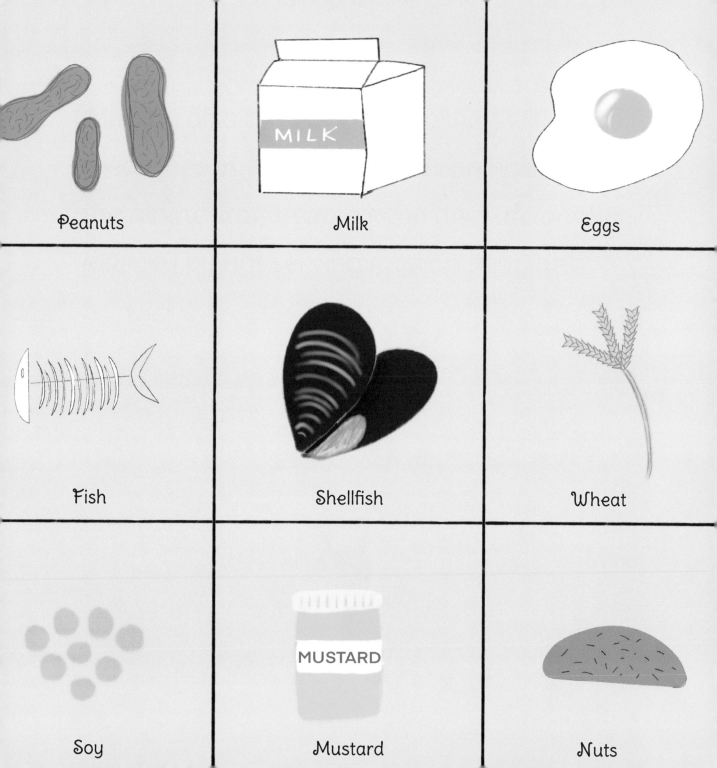

Peanuts

Milk

Eggs

Fish

Shellfish

Wheat

Soy

Mustard

Nuts

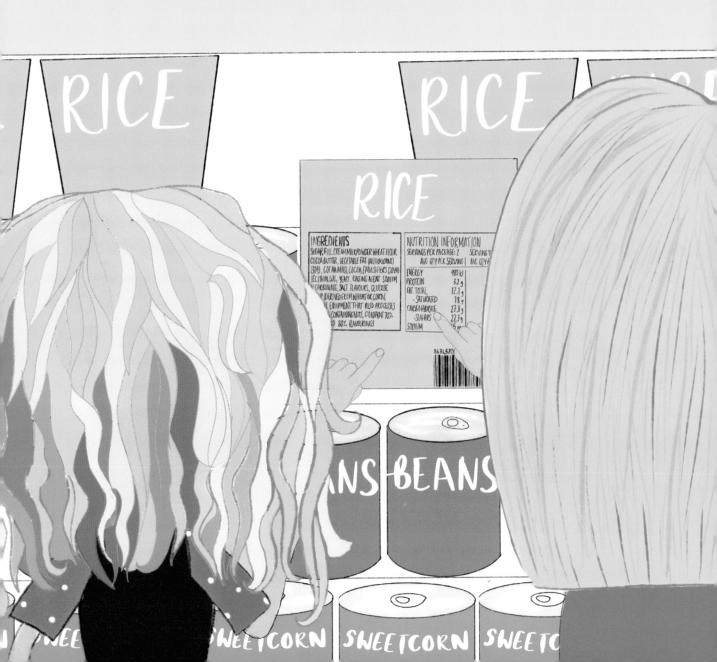

To stay healthy and safe Matilda has to check food labels with her mum. She must not take food off anyone without checking it first.

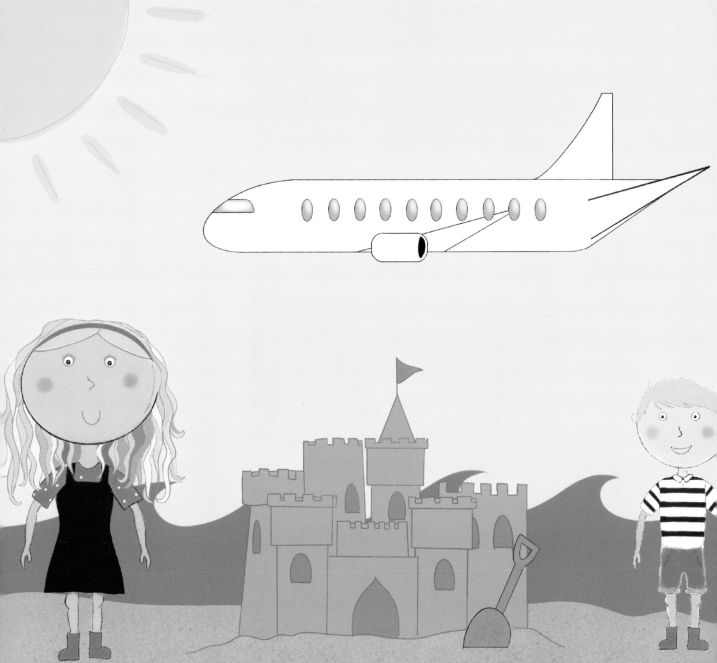

Matilda also carries a special bag with her medicines in. When she goes on holiday the airline staff help to keep her safe on the journey by not serving nuts on the plane

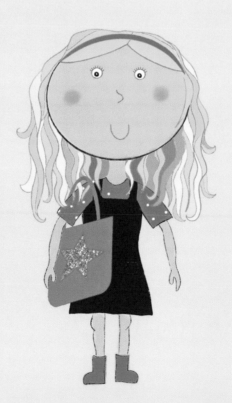

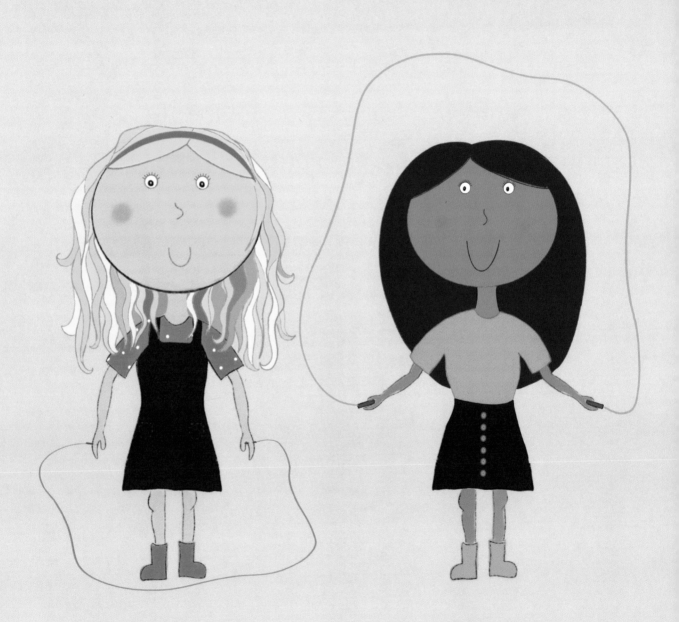

Matilda can still have lots of fun with her best friend Leila. Leila doesn't have a food allergy but she understands all about Matilda's allergy and how to help keep her safe.

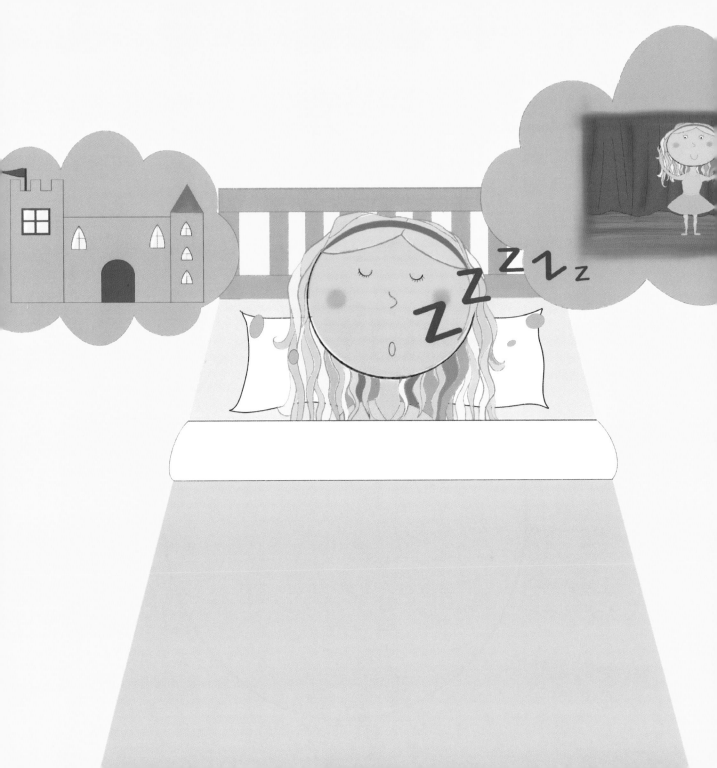

So that's a little bit about Matilda and her allergy. Matilda is allergy aware; she knows food needs to be checked and she carries her special medicine wherever she goes. She wants to help more people become allergy aware so that other children with allergies are even safer. Matilda dreams of having more amazing adventures. After all, Matilda loves being Matilda.

I am Allergy Aware

Draw yourself in the circle
to show that you are Allergy Aware

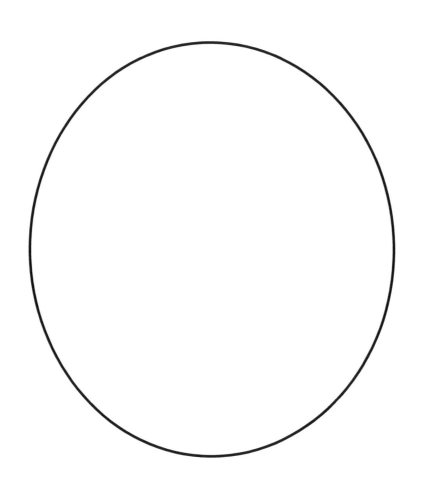

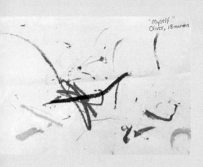

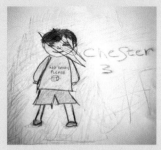

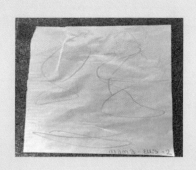

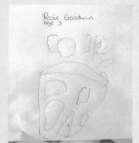

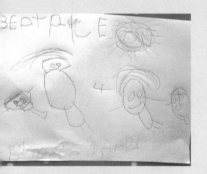

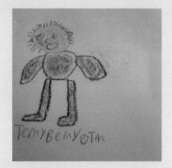

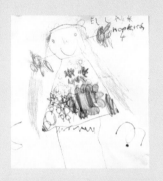

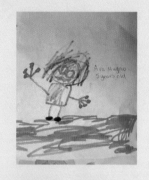

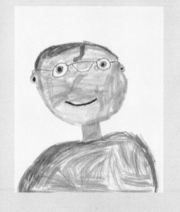

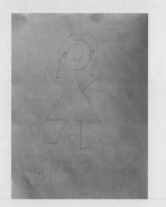

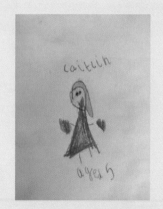

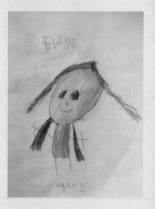

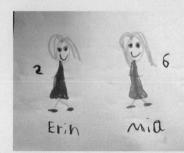

We have allergies too

Lightning Source UK Ltd.
Milton Keynes UK
UKIC012338040920
369384UK00005B/103